# Seven Effective Strategies For Getting into the Best Shape of Your Life

## Barry Nashen

# Introduction

Imagine this: You're in the best shape of your life. Lately, people you know well, and even people you barely know at all, have been asking you for advice about how they, too, can get into fantastic shape. They are asking you to reveal your secret formula. Is this a dream, or can you make it a reality?

One morning last week I woke up and realized that this fantasy is actually my life story! Not only this, I know and understand how you can make this dream your reality, too. I decided to write it all down and reveal to you what is standing between the present you and the future you. The present you, well, you know this character all too well. The future you is that individual that other people admire, partly because you look great and you feel awesome.

It's true, most of us want to get into great shape and feel wonderful. Yet according to a recent study published in *The Lancet*, the majority of us are out of shape, suffer too often from fatigue and sleep poorly. Many of us wake up mornings feeling as though we need more sleep. In fact, if not for the alarm clock ringing in the morning, we would sleep another hour or more.

Why is this? If we tell ourselves that we want to go to the gym to take cardio classes or swim or lift weights then why aren't we doing so? If we plan to run or cycle on weekends when we have ample time, then why aren't we following through? When we start a fitness program, why do we give up after a few weeks or months? Did you know that two thirds of adults who make New Year's resolutions have set fitness goals as part of their resolution? Yet nearly half of those who gave up before reaching their fitness resolution goal did so within six weeks, according to a recent online study conducted by Harris Interactive. Not only are we evidently abandoning our fitness resolution but we are doing it with haste!

If you are like most people you may see yourself falling into this same frustrating pattern. If so, this book is for you. You are about to read about seven proven and effective strategies for getting into the best shape of your life, for feeling wonderful, energetic and enthusiastic thanks to your own success, personal improvement and accomplishments. Furthermore, once you have achieved your goals, you can use these same strategies to maintain your new fitness level or even to surpass it when you choose to do so.

Whether you decide that it is time to lose weight, or to add lean muscle, or to run a road race and cross the finish line, or to simply feel wonderful and fit, any of these seven strategies will propel you forward to succeed and ultimately to keep your new fitness level for life. The old you will remain in your past. The new you will be yours to enjoy forever!

Why seven strategies? Let me explain. What is lacking in nearly all fitness programs is the one critical ingredient on which success depends: Motivation. If you are reading this book, you already have the required motivation to start a fitness program; however we all need motivation to stick to the program and to enjoy it, too. Without motivation, everybody will find any of a hundred reasons to skip a workout. You probably already know the excuses that people tell themselves – your spouse needs you to be elsewhere, your kids need rides to soccer practice or piano lessons, you have to work late, you're tired, your friends want you to join them for happy hour drinks, or you didn't sleep enough last night and you feel drained. The list is long! Do you ever wonder why something else, anything else, suddenly becomes more important to do than what you had intended? This is not from bad luck or poor planning. Without appropriate motivation, our unconscious minds will always protect us from the risk of failure or the risk of exhaustion or the risk of embarrassment and present one or two appealing alternatives to our conscious minds just in the nick of time. You can always blame the demanding boss, or your loving spouse, or your well-intentioned friends for your missed workout.

We can all agree that different people require different strategies for success. Depending on our personal preferences, experiences and our own unique DNA, a strategy that works wonders for John may fail miserably for Jane. While reading about the seven unique strategies for getting and staying motivated, each of you will be naturally attracted to two or three of them. Just as you may have a favorite food or a favorite beer or wine, you will find that two or three of these strategies make sense to you, personally, at a deep level. Then, simply pick these and use them. You will probably surprise yourself that while all previous attempts to get into great shape have failed, this time you are persevering and more importantly that you are enjoying the training. Now your unconscious mind will ensure that your workouts are indeed your priority and will always clear a path for you to keep to a schedule. The expected results of great health, more energy, deeper sleep, and feeling wonderful will always trump other competing offers vying for your time and attention. Such is the promise of this book. Discover the motivation that works for you and claim what is rightfully yours: Feeling wonderful and achieving the level of fitness that you deserve!

Many people ask how often they must train. Are three days a week enough, or too much, or too little? The answer is, it depends on your fitness goals. Some years ago I saw a pamphlet from a fitness organization that had three pictures on the front panel, one under the other, of essentially the same person. The first picture showed the person in pretty fine form, a look that most of us would be happy to have; to the right of the picture, "2 days per week" was written. However, the second photo showed who we often see on the cover of a fitness magazine; to the right of the photo, "4 days per week" was printed. Can you guess the rest? The third image showed a bodybuilder with bulging muscles; to the right of the image, "6 days per week" was printed.

The images remain etched into my memory after these many years as they continue to remind me that what we get out of our training efforts is directly proportional to what we put in. For those of you who are now planning to finally get into shape, to feel great, and most importantly to maintain this new level of fitness for life, why not start with a training schedule of three days per week? You can always adjust this later as you see and feel the results. For instance, you may choose to increase the frequency that you decide to do some physical activities.

Another popular question asked is what training is required? Is walking sufficient or do we have to become runners or swimmers or weightlifters? Can't we just play tennis or golf twice a week? There is no magic in the answer: To get into the best shape of our lives and feel wonderful, it is essential that we engage in two kinds of activities on an ongoing basis:

1.  We burn calories
2.  We stress or load our muscles

If your fitness goal is endurance-based, then your focus may be on running, cycling or swimming, to name just three popular sports. In this case, I recommend to mix in a weight training, pilates or yoga class once a week. On the other hand, if your fitness goal is strength-oriented, then your focus will be on weight training. In this case, I recommend to mix in a weekly run or Zumba class.

Many fitness centers offer boot camps or cross-fit programs. These classes combine both calorie burning and muscle loading at once and are also very successful methods of getting into the best shape of your life.

The human body is designed to be in motion. It is most content and most healthy when it performs physical activity regularly. The latest research bears out this fact as is reported routinely in a variety of popular magazines and scientific papers. The World Health Organization (WHO) asserts that physical inactivity constitutes the fourth leading cause of death globally.

You deserve to feel fantastic. The purpose of this book is to outline in detail seven strategies proven to be successful at keeping yourself motivated to get into the best shape of your life and feel great!

Let's get started...

# Strategy One: Set a specific and clear goal

Strategy One is essential to your success. I highly recommended that you choose to employ this first strategy and then consider adding any one or two of the other strategies that excite you. As I will explain in a moment, this concept by itself may be all you need to align your actions with your objective. It is both powerful and magical in how this strategy persistently and quietly reprograms your unconscious mind to focus on success. You will not even be aware consciously of what is going on, but deep inside your mind your goal is in laser focus.

Your goal needs to have four simple components to get you on the right path: it must be specific, clear, realistic and challenging. Let me explain these last two components first.

Successful people routinely set goals for themselves. But not just any goal, they set difficult, challenging goals. It is too easy to abandon an everyday or average objective when time is tight or the going gets tough. How many times have you promised yourself to do something seemingly simple but you still managed to avoid following through? As an example, say you decide that you want to run a 5 km race in under 30 minutes. You know you can do it. Somebody at your office has done it, or one of your friends. Wouldn't you feel twice as proud if you decided, instead, to run a 5 km race in under 25 minutes? This new goal may even scare you as you are not even sure you will succeed! But this is exactly why this ingredient is critical. Your goal must be difficult enough that you feel challenged to go for it. A goal that is too easy is no goal at all. And one that is too difficult will frustrate and discourage you from giving 100% to the effort. Consider your own experiences with some personal or professional projects that you have managed in the past and realize that the easy ones are the most forgettable, while the very hardest ones were a waste of your time as success was never actually within your grasp.

To explain all four components of goal setting in real terms, here are some choice examples of excellent goals vs. inadequate goals:

Running. Assuming that 5 km is both realistic and challenging for you:
Inadequate: I want to run in a 5-km race.
Excellent: I want to run a 5-km race in under 25 minutes by the end of May.

Swimming. Assuming that swimming 1,500 meters is both realistic and challenging for you:
Inadequate goal: I want to swim better.
Excellent goal: I want to swim 1,500 meters in under 30 minutes by the end of August.

Weight loss. Assuming that losing 40 pounds is both realistic and challenging for you:
Inadequate: I want to lose some weight.
Excellent: I want to lose 40 pounds in the next six months.

Cycling. Assuming that 50 km (or 30 miles) is both realistic and challenging for you:
Inadequate: I want to cycle faster.

Excellent: I want to cycle 50 km (or 30 miles) in under two hours by the first day of July.

Weight training. Assuming that the bench press is on your mind:
Inadequate: I want to bench 185 pounds.
Excellent: I want to bench 6 reps at 185 pounds within four months.

Let's explore the psychology behind goal setting. Our brains sift through billions of bits of data at any given moment. And somehow, so we don't short circuit, we have to organize that information. This is where the Reticular Activating System (RAS) comes along. According to the *Textbook of Clinical Neurology*, the RAS is a bundle of nerves in our brains that filters out unnecessary information so the important stuff gets through.

The RAS is the reason that when you decide on buying a certain model car, you suddenly start seeing it everywhere. It's why you can tune out a crowd full of talking people, yet suddenly become alert when someone in that same crowd speaks your name.

Your RAS takes what you focus on and creates a filter for it. It then sifts through the data and presents only the fragments that are important to you. All of this happens without you noticing. The RAS programs itself to work in your favor without you actively doing anything. You may be nodding your head in agreement at this moment as you think of an experience that you have had in the past week or two that now suddenly makes sense.

In the same way, the RAS seeks information that validates your beliefs. It filters the world through the parameters you give it, and your beliefs shape those parameters. If you think you are bad at giving speeches, you probably will be. If you believe you deserve to get into the best shape of your life, you most likely will. Your RAS helps you see what you want to see and in doing so, influences your actions. Take ten seconds to reread the last sentence.

Some people suggest that you can train your RAS by taking your unconscious thoughts and marrying them to your conscious thoughts. They call it "setting your intent." This basically means that if you focus hard on your goals, your RAS will reveal the people, information and opportunities that help you achieve them.

A technique exists which you can implement that does in fact train your RAS and it is called SMARTER goals. You can follow my fitness-oriented version right here. I have successfully employed it many times with many people. It will certainly work for you, too! When you are ready to install SMARTER goals in your mind, first set aside about 20 minutes to properly focus on the answers to the upcoming questions and the exercise that follows. It is so important to understand these questions, think carefully about your answers and write them down on a sheet of paper. Many psychologists recommend that you tape this completed sheet of questions and answers to your fridge as a daily reminder.

The simple act of writing down a goal is enough to program ourselves to behave accordingly. If you have personal integrity, then all the parts of your mind will unconsciously conspire to keep your promise, to act in a way that your fitness goal will be realized. Your priorities are rearranged in the back of your mind so that the time you need to train will magically become available.

Let's get started.

1. State your goal in clear, specific and positive terms. What do you want precisely?
2. Your goal must be measureable in terms of sensory experience. How will you know you have achieved this outcome; what will you see, hear and feel when you have achieved it?
3. Do you believe that your goal is actually achievable now?
4. Are you in control of doing everything necessary to achieve this outcome? A well-formed goal cannot be dependent on the actions of another person or situation.
5. By when exactly are you committed to having achieved this outcome? When will you take the next step?
6. Examine the outcome in relation to all the key areas of life, such as: work, relationships, health, emotional well-being, etc. Keep these areas in mind as you explore the following questions:
   What will you gain by doing it?
   What will you lose by not doing it?
7. Ask results-oriented questions:
   Why do you want to get into the best shape of your life?

What will change for you?
What would be the consequences of not getting into the best shape of your life?

And now it is time for the fun exercise. It may seem silly when you read the instructions. You may say to yourself, "Sure, I'll do it later." However you may react, invest five minutes and enjoy this exercise now. I always receive amazing feedback from people after performing this experiment. Once you have read these instructions, close your eyes and do it.

Sit comfortably, undisturbed by kids, television, etc., and close your eyes:

Picture yourself in the future, once you have attained your outcome, getting into the best shape of your life.

1. Imagine how you will look, see yourself standing tall in the mirror, as others will be seeing you. If you are smiling proudly at your fit body looking back at you from the other side of the mirror, then see yourself smiling. Turn yourself to see your body in profile and enjoy how great you look. You are gazing at the future you.

2. Imagine what you will hear. What are your friends and family saying, are they complimenting your new look? What are others asking you, for advice on getting themselves into great shape, too?

3. Now imagine how you feel in your new fit-for-life body. Do you feel wonderful? Powerful like Superman or Wonder Woman? Are you thrilled? Are you proud? Feel these feelings now as you imagine yourself in the future and enjoy them for a few minutes. These

fantastic feelings are yours to enjoy now as you imagine your future self.

This completes the SMARTER goals exercise. If you can't remember the instructions in the above paragraph, ask somebody to read them to you while your eyes are closed which will enable you to enjoy the experience with more intensity.

After reading and understanding goal setting, the popular Law of Attraction doesn't seem so mystical. Focus on the bad things and you will invite negativity into your life. Focus on the good things and they will come to you, because your brain is seeking them out. It's not magic, it's your Reticular Activating System influencing the world you see around you.

# Strategy Two: Enlist a friend

Social scientists know that humans are social beings. Most of us have a few close relationships, with our partners, our families and our friends. Research proves that, on average, we are happiest when we are sharing experiences with others. We become more engaged, more motivated and in the case of physical activities we are also often more competitive. A healthy competitive spirit between friends and acquaintances is a strong motivator to push ourselves.

A study published in the scientific journal *Nature Communications* found that friends have a major influence on a person's exercise routine. The study found that not only are we inspired by our friends to get out and exercise, but we also display our competitive streak by wanting to outperform their accomplishments. When your friend runs longer or faster, you want to, also. When your friend lifts heavier weight, you are motivated to do the same.

Strategy Two for success to get into the best shape of your life is to train or do your workouts with a friend. You may be willing to let yourself down by skipping a workout, but nobody wants to let down a friend. You are accountable to your training partner and he or she is counting on you to show up on schedule for your workout without fail, just as you expect your friend to arrive on time as well, ready to enjoy your time together, even as you perspire.

Picture this: you're in a car driving somewhere on a frigid cold, sub-zero, winter evening. Or, if you prefer, it's a sunny, blistering hot 100 degrees day. In either case, you look outside and see two friends running together, smiling and chatting, evidently oblivious to the very uncomfortable weather conditions. You are probably wondering, why would they do this?

Here's the answer: Friends support each other. Neither one wants to bail and let down the other. Chatting for an hour, while running, is a huge distraction from the day's problems and certainly from the extreme temperatures. And remember the terrific satisfaction they will both earn for having persevered in these challenging conditions. They have both earned bragging rights.

There are so many great reasons for training with a friend. Here are my favorites:

1. **You push each other.** If your workout partner is stronger or faster than you, you'll be more likely to push the envelope and exceed your self-imposed limitations. I say "self-imposed' because I have heard countless times a person maintaining that running any faster than X or lifting a weight heavier than Y was impossible. The very short phrase, "I can't," is usually what I hear. She has imposed on herself the limitation of X or he has imposed on himself the constraint of Y. Rest assured that there are no real barriers, only imaginary ones. Training with a friend is frequently all it takes to punch through your previously held, imaginary obstacle. A wager with your partner may be the extra kick that allows you to excel. Remember, you are now getting into the best shape of your life, so you can expect to continually bust

through the envelope of possibilities. The first time that you exceed a previously held self-limiting belief is all the proof you need that you had until then imposed the restriction on yourself, for no valid reason. From that time forward and for the rest of your life, you will profoundly understand that there are no limitations. Other people may tell you that you cannot achieve X or Y, but you will know otherwise.

2. **Training is more fun.** Many beginners are shy to try something new in the gym, like a newfangled piece of equipment, either for strength training or for a cardio workout. Few people however are intimidated when doing something novel with a friend. At the least you will have a laugh together if you end up facing the wrong way when trying the latest machine for the first time. In addition, in the case of weight training, you will feel more motivated to adding extra weight to your routine if you know that your partner will spot you. If the extra weight is indeed too much during your set, your friend will keep you from hurting yourself. Or you can try different exercises that you cannot do alone, like throwing a ball back and forth while doing sit-ups. How about racing each other around a track, or, who can run the farthest in 60 seconds, a challenge given or received in the middle of a run with your friend?

3. **Work out longer.** Time flies when you're having fun or being distracted. Having someone to chat with between sets at the gym or during a run does make time fly. In these cases you have the opportunity to train 15, 20 or even 30 minutes longer without really being aware of the extra period spent exercising. But your body will definitely benefit by the additional minutes. In the case of weight training, you will have spent more minutes with your muscles under load, which translates into bigger gains in less time. In the case of running or swimming or cycling, you will be expanding your capacity for endurance. Both stronger muscles and greater endurance affect all aspects of your life, not just your fitness level. You may suddenly find yourself feeling like Superman or Wonder Woman when you least expect it or when you most need it.

4. **Train together and stay together.** It's no secret that getting buff helps you out in the bedroom thanks to a boost in your strength, endurance and flexibility — but a sweat session also has more immediate effects. "Endorphins from exercise give you an adrenaline rush that boosts arousal," says Terri Orbuch, a marriage researcher and author. Activities that get your heart rate up, like running or biking, are guaranteed to have a positive effect on desire. Any kind of arousal rush will be transferred to your romantic partner and add passion to your relationship.

Your brain will simply associate feeling great with your partner. You may find yourself feeling aroused by your partner even when you are not running or biking. Everybody wins in this scenario.

5. **Recover together.** There's nothing worse than undoing all your hard work at the gym by eating unhealthy afterwards. You and your friend will encourage each other to go out for a healthy post-exercise meal or snack after training together to chat. There's nothing wrong with sometimes going to a bar or lounge for a glass of wine or beer as long as you limit the calories consumed. Knowing that you intend to go out for a drink with your friend once a week or twice a month will likely make the workout on that night even more satisfying.

# Strategy Three: Join a gym and socialize

We lead busy lives. Between work responsibilities, family commitments and losing valuable time commuting to and from work, we often have no time left over to nurture friendships. Sadly, we may even wake up one day and realize that we no longer have any close friends. Everybody else is suffering from the very same constraints and has become caught up in their own realities of family and work with little free time of their own. Life was a lot simpler when we were students, surrounded by our best friends, learning together, scheming together and having the most fun. Even after graduating, but before the kids arrived in our lives, we always had time for our friends. Here's some good news: It's not too late to recreate the care-free, school-age environment that we are now recalling. If you join a running club, a swim team or a gym, open your eyes to the possibility of not only completing your workouts but also of making new friends. Your new friends will have similar goals as you so why not combine your regular workouts with socializing, learning about new ideas and enjoying novel conversations with people that have similar fitness objectives, but different life experiences than yourself?

Research by Nicholas Christakis at Yale University found that relationships are the number one promoter of happiness in life. A bigger network leads to bigger happiness, according to the Yale study. When friends of friends become happier, it ripples through the social circle. Their happiness can affect yours. There are other collateral benefits to a bigger network to consider. "You are the average of the five people that you spend the most time with," a quote attributed most often to motivational speaker Jim Rohn. When it comes to relationships, we are greatly influenced — whether we like it or not — by those closest to us. It affects our way of thinking, our self-esteem, and our decisions.

My argument is clear-cut. Without making an effort to make new friends at the gym, you will almost certainly do so anyway; either in the locker room thanks to your chatty neighbor, in the weight room when somebody is waiting to use your station or bench, or more naturally if you join a swim team or a running club. These new friends will likely have different life experiences than yours. It is probable that, by chance, new ideas, new business or networking opportunities, or new introductions will result, as long as you are open to the possibility. Ultimately, you may end up with a new, more promising job, or a new business partner, or even a new romantic partner. All of these outcomes are side benefits of your primary decision to get into the best shape of your life. Knowing that you will be seeing friendly faces, having novel conversations, all while working towards your goal is superb motivation to sticking to your workout schedule.

Conversely, a weak social circle is bad for your health. According to research from Brigham Young University, not having enough friends is the same risk factor as smoking 15 cigarettes a day. Most of us will not find these discoveries so outrageous. When we look around at our acquaintances and work colleagues, it is easy to acknowledge that the happier people are usually the same individuals who are most popular, having large networks of friends. Once new friendships are forged at the gym, running club or cycling group, it will suddenly and naturally be a pleasure and not a chore to work out regularly. You may even find yourself slipping in an additional workout some weeks rather than concocting excuses for missing one.

At every level, physical and neural, locations get linked to memories. Places get associated with the type of activity that occurs there, and the pattern can be nearly impossible to break. The link between location and thought explains why many of us cannot work from home and need to go to a workplace, the office, in order to work productively. At home, we are not used to working and we find ourselves distracted by the same things that we would normally do around the house. Those neural associations and memory traces are not the ones that you want to activate. The ones that you do want to activate – working out, perspiring, training – can be consistently found at the gym. Most everybody agrees on the satisfaction they get after a hard workout and a refreshing shower. Once this feeling of satisfaction is embedded in your mind as being linked to the gym or running club or swimming pool, you will naturally and unconsciously feel happy about your training program. This process only takes about three workouts. Imagine, after your first week at the gym, it will suddenly feel pleasurable to be heading to your workout. This is simply human nature and it will happen to you, too. What better motivation to continuing with your program and achieving your fitness goal than by feeling happy to put in the effort?

If you haven't been to the gym in a while, or if you have never joined a gym until now, here is a great idea: On your first visit, arrange for a trainer or coach to explain the options that the gym offers. Understand the different machines used in weight training and those used in aerobic activities. Things have changed a lot in the past decade. Many treadmills and stationary bicycles now have big color screens that can offer you a choice of workouts. You can connect your headphones or earbuds, whether wired or wireless, to the display if you prefer to watch the news or your favorite show, or browse the Internet while engaged in your workout.

There are likely three or four different cycling machines, five or six different running machines, some of them engaging your arms as well. One variety is designed to have zero impact so you can run with no risk of injury to your knees. Rowing machines will stress your arms, abs, back and legs with every stroke. There are stairmasters, stairclimbers and never-ending ladders to climb at different speeds and intensities. Boxing classes have become popular, pilates remains in vogue and boot camps are popping up at many gyms. Inform yourself what your gym has to offer and integrate one or more of these options into your training program. It is always a smart idea to mix up your primary training routine with other, different complementary routines. We call it cross-training and it wakes up those muscles that may not otherwise be stressed in your usual program.

Novel classes or machines motivate you as you strive to improve your fitness level. Group classes are fun for most people. You can chat with people nearby before and after your class. During the class, the energy in the room is contagious, the music is upbeat, and the instructor is inspiring. Remember, in a group class, you want to be an overachiever. When you push yourself to your limit, your limit expands. As a rule, then, always be pushing yourself to your limit in a group class. Most people cruise through these classes with little benefit. You see them after months and even years with zero change in their fitness levels. There is no advantage to comparing your output or effort with these average people. Instead, give the others in the class good reason for trying to keep up with you.

As I emphasized in the previous paragraph, when you push yourself to your limit, your limit expands. Essentially, you find yourself in a virtuous circle as you get stronger and your endurance increases. This is especially true in boot camp-style classes as you are working your muscles and your cardiovascular system all at once. It bears repeating that when you train at the gym, most people are on auto-pilot, often spending more time on their phones than working out. You want to maximize your precious free time and this means training hard at the gym. Training hard does not imply that you want to kill yourself so that you can barely drag your beat-up body to the locker room after your workout. It does mean that you have perspired, your heart rate has increased, your muscles are tired, and counterintuitively you feel great.

You always want to feel great after exercising. It is a primary motivator to persist, which naturally results in a continual and steady improvement in your strength and endurance. If you are dead tired after training or if fatigue continues even after adequate rest, then you are likely overtraining. If you feel nothing after your workouts, then you are probably undertraining. In either case, you failed to maximize your time spent at the gym. Overtraining can be dangerous for your health as other problems will likely follow, such as increased incidence of injury and higher susceptibility to infections. Undertraining is simply a waste of your time, isn't it? It may be alright for others, but not for you.

# Strategy Four: Reward yourself

Many people have heard or read about the experiments of Ivan Pavlov, performed at the end of the nineteenth century. In fact, he was awarded the Nobel Prize in 1904 for his work. Pavlov demonstrated that a physical cue (in his experiment it was a sound, however it can just as easily be something visual or a smell or a general location) could eventually elicit the same response as an actual reward. So, the story goes, he would ring a bell and then present his dogs with food. Naturally, at the sight of the food, the dogs would salivate. But soon enough, and this is the shocking truth, the dogs began to salivate at the sound of the bell itself, before any sight or smell of food. The bell triggered the anticipation of the food and with it, the physical reaction.

This has come to be known as classical conditioning. It is not a trick; it is simply how the mind works. In a more human example, many of us will suddenly and automatically smile and feel wonderful when passing in front of a bakery. The smell of freshly baked breads elicits memories of our coming home from school to be greeted by these same smells when our mothers or grandmothers were busily baking our favorite treats.

How can we take advantage of this conditioning to help us to remain motivated in our goal of getting into the best shape of our lives? The answer is straightforward. After every workout treat yourself. You only earn this reward by completing the workout. Before long your mind will associate the workout with the treat. That is, your workout will feel more and more enjoyable. In fact, the workout itself will elicit the same pleasure as the reward does.

What kind of reward? It may be one of your favourite indulgences, like an ice cream, or relaxing in the sauna (if your gym or home has one), or a cold beer or glass of wine for no other reason at all. You've earned the treat, so enjoy it. The more you enjoy the reward, the more you will enjoy the workout. Of course, if food or beverage is your chosen prize, ensure that its portion size matches the workout effort. In time, you will realize that becoming fit and feeling great is its own reward. Until then, classical conditioning is an effortless tool to use and will always work for you. It is simply human nature.

Another strategy using rewards may be better suited. Rather than indulging yourself after every workout, create a much bigger and more enticing reward once your ultimate goal has been achieved. I have a friend who is crazy for soccer, what Europeans call football. His reward for achieving his training goal was to travel to the city hosting the World Cup the next year and spend the better part of a week attending as many matches as possible. This reward was a luxury that he never imagined he could arrange for all the usual reasons of finances, time off from work, time away from his family, etc. However once he had it in his mind to reward himself, you can guess that he never missed a workout.

As an example, say you have challenged yourself to run a marathon. That's 26 miles, or 42 kilometers, of running with very few, if any, breaks from the punishing, tiring ordeal of your feet pounding the pavement. Most large cities around the world host an annual marathon whose circuits often pass through the most picturesque or historical parts of town. Each event will attract thousands of willing participants where only a small fraction are elite runners. The greater majority are regular folks who have chosen to challenge themselves by completing the full course without failure. Some people have specific targets, such as running a four-hour marathon, others have the goal of simply crossing the finish line, with no time target at all. Why not run yours in another country?

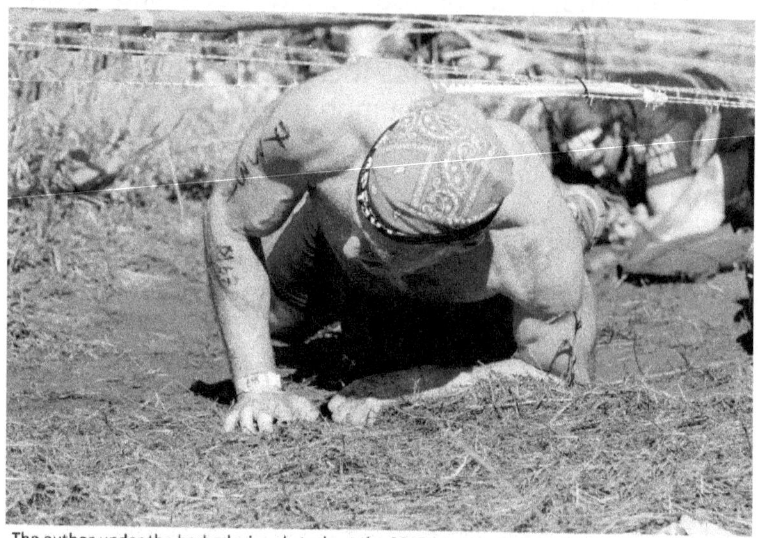
The author under the barbed wire obstacle at the 2015 Montreal Spartan Beast

I have a friend who wanted to enter a body-building competition before his 50th birthday. He needed to get into great shape, engage a coach to learn the poses and modify his nutritional intake. It's a big ordeal so he created a big reward for himself (and for his family, who were cheerleading from the sidelines).

He couldn't imagine letting his family down so his motivation was always high even though he had nearly a year of hard work ahead of him before he could compete. Can you imagine letting your family down – I doubt it very much?

Your workout goal may be less spectacular: lose 25 pounds; learn to swim; bench press your weight; run a 5-km race; cycle 30 miles; the list is endless. Once you have set your goal that you believe you can achieve within six to twelve months of training, then create your just reward.

Everybody loves rewards but there is some psychology behind this. In Mihaly Csikszentmihalyi's ground-breaking book, *Flow: The Psychology of Optimal Experience*, he outlines his theory that people are happiest when they are in a state of flow — a state of concentration or complete absorption with the activity at hand and the situation. It is a state in which people are so involved in an activity that nothing else seems to matter. The idea of flow is identical to the feeling of being *in the zone* or *in the groove*. The flow state is an optimal state of *intrinsic motivation*, where the person is fully immersed in what he or she is doing. This is a perception everyone has at times, characterized by a feeling of great absorption, engagement, fulfillment, and skill — and during which temporal concerns (time, food, ego-self, etc.) are typically ignored.

Csikszentmihályi characterized nine component states of achieving flow. The three components that interest us are "challenge-skill balance, clarity of goals, and immediate and unambiguous feedback." There is no better way of being motivated into getting into the best shape of your life than by getting into the flow state during every workout. And we do this by having challenges in line with our inherent skills, by having clear goals (ultimately leading to our earned reward), and by having feedback which informs us that we are slowly but surely improving and thus approaching our goal.

Challenge-skill balance: When we set a goal and totally immerse ourselves in it, we not only experience a temporary euphoric state of mind as we are totally involved in the process, but our self-esteem rises as we move closer to achieving our goal. Not only this, but that wonderful sense of well-being and lifted self-esteem stay with us for quite some time. But there is one distinct critical key if we want to ensure our success: The goals that we set for ourselves must be difficult. They must make us struggle in order to have the euphoric drug-like effect. However one must have the confidence in one's ability to complete the challenge, as difficult as it may be.

Clarity of goals: We have discussed this component in detail in Strategy One. To briefly recap, a clear set of goals and progress add direction and structure to the task. The task is today's workout program. There is a saying, "you can't manage what you can't measure." Creating a clear goal allows you to measure your progress.

Immediate and unambiguous feedback: Today's workout must have clear and immediate feedback. This will help you to negotiate any changing demands and allows you to adjust your performance to maintain the flow state. Here is a simple example: Your plan was to run a mile on the track in 7 minutes, four times.

On the first mile, you could barely make it in 7:30. The second mile had similar results. Before killing yourself on the third mile, acknowledge that today's goal is too difficult. Maybe there is a wind, or it is too humid, or you had an argument with your boss, and your running has been compromised. To remain in the flow state, adjust your goal, aim for 7:30 for your third and fourth miles.

# Strategy Five: Hire a coach

A fitness coach works with you on developing a positive mindset, helps set realistic and actionable goals, and strives to keep you motivated and accountable in the process. Sounds perfect, right? Personal coaching sessions could be a great way to fire up your fitness program, and importantly, transform your attitude about physical activity. If you are the kind of person that needs a push from time to time, then keep reading. Engaging a coach or trainer may be your best strategy for getting into the best shape of your life.

A good personal fitness trainer is an individual with expert knowledge across a large array of fitness topics and exercise types, especially the kind of training that meets your personal objectives. A personal trainer with this type of knowledge and experience is what you are looking for. A knowledgeable personal fitness trainer will have specific insight related to a multitude of fitness programs, techniques and physical injuries and/or limitations.

In fact, a personal fitness trainer will most likely be able to guide you step-by-step through a fitness program that is specifically designed to meet your needs and goals. In so doing, a personal trainer may be able to assist you in maximizing your efforts and obtaining your specific goals at a rate quicker than if you had taken your personal fitness journey alone.

The most obvious benefit you will gain from hiring a personal fitness trainer is his or her specific knowledge and expertise about health, fitness and mental well-being. However, it may be a challenge to find an instructor that is well-versed in all of the aspects associated with good health. You may have to experiment with several trainers before you find the one that works best for you. Personal fitness trainers are just like any other service-oriented profession. That is, you may have to steer through a few personal trainers before you find the one that understands you best. Establishing rapport with your coach is essential to keeping you motivated to continue on the program that you both agree to. If you do not admire your coach or if you do not look forward to your next workout with him or her, it is time to look around for a replacement. I cannot overemphasize the importance for having a strong rapport with your personal trainer as he or she is in the absolute best position to influence you to never give up and to continue prioritizing your training program.

However, once you have found a knowledgeable personal fitness trainer that you admire and enjoy working with, he or she will be able to provide you with expert knowledge related specifically to your body and the best way to go about obtaining your personal fitness goals. This approach will save you an enormous amount of time, minimize your frustration due to trial and error, and jumpstart your fitness program.

In addition, a personal fitness trainer will be able to maximize your results and minimize the time you spend working out, since you will be performing a fitness program that he or she has specifically designed to meet your unique needs and goals. Also, a personal trainer will be able to periodically modify your workout routine to ensure that your body is in a continual state of development and that you are consistently moving closer to achieving your personal fitness goals. Remember, you must be exercising at or near your limit in order to expand your endurance and get stronger. A great trainer will ensure that this is the case during your sessions together.

A huge benefit derived from hiring a personal fitness trainer is motivation. Your instructor will expect that you show up to perform all of your scheduled workouts, and will hold you accountable when you do not. In addition, personal trainers will also provide you with motivation when you are actually working out. This will include pushing you to your physical and mental limits so that they assist you in maximizing the efficiency of your workout time and creating an environment where you are able to achieve your personal fitness goals in the shortest time possible.

At times, it may seem like your personal fitness trainer is pushing you – aggressively – and that they are not as easy-going as when your training relationship began. This is normal, as they truly have your personal health and well-being in mind as their top priority. They only succeed when you thrive.

An experienced trainer will quickly understand your strengths and weaknesses. He will understand the training goal that you have established for yourself. He will create a training program to ensure your success, improve your technique, monitor your progress and then modify your program to maintain a steady improvement. If your instructor is not accomplishing these tasks, or if your gains are appearing too slowly, then start searching for a new coach. Your time is precious. Every hour that you invest in yourself should contribute to your achieving the goal that you have established for yourself. Other people may choose to squander their training efforts with wasteful distractions or poor technique, but not you.

Progress is a great motivator. It's the best kind of feedback that you can receive. It is impartial and does not require any cheering from another person. Smart coaches believe that your own personal progress is its own reward whereas improving your performance solely for the approval of another person will quickly lose its value. Allow me to repeat this point: It is always nice to hear our coach praise us for an achievement attained but true satisfaction can only come from within. Achieving both your short term and long term goals is its own reward.

# Strategy Six: Wear Technology

Some people are naturally motivated to excel by receiving immediate and detailed feedback about their physical efforts and resulting statistics. If this describes you, then you're in luck. There are now a number of devices that fit into the class of products called wearable technology. There are two types of devices that you can choose from and either one will provide you with the exercise details that you may be craving for.

You probably already own one of them: Your smartphone. You can download an app to your smartphone, such as the ever-popular application, Strava. As long as you carry the phone with you, it will track your every move. Depending on the activity that you select, it will measure your steps, your speed, your distance, changes in elevation or any number of other metrics that pertain to your activity. Even hikers, skiers, kayakers and weightlifters enjoy tracking their activities and keeping training logs.

Or, you can purchase a physical tracking device, such as Fitbit or Garmin, which you simply wear on your wrist. It collects roughly the same information as the smartphone app (as well as record your sleep pattern if you wish) and there is no requirement to carry or even to own a smartphone. The wristband will collect the statistics that matter to you, eventually synchronizing with your smartphone, your smartwatch or your computer and provide you the feedback that interests you.

Real-time monitoring of your progress is a big boost for many athletes and therefore a strong motivator. Even the smallest improvements in your training will be made obvious, providing you with reasons to pat yourself on the back as you move forward toward your fitness goal. Many of the wearables simultaneously monitor your heart rate which adds to the information and statistics that are reported back to you once synchronized. This added data can be used to calculate calories burned during your workout which many people like to monitor, in particular for those who are planning on losing weight as a result of their training program. I know someone who feels the he must burn 4,000 calories per week while exercising. We can debate the benefits of this target but in his case it is a great motivator to always be wearing his fitness device when training and track his weekly progress to the magic 4,000 calorie mark.

As a side note, some studies have shown that many people, when wearing a fitness tracking device, view their workouts less like a chore and more like a game or fun activity. Like any captivating game, just a tap or click and you immediately see data which maps out your progress. If your average speed during a run or bike ride climbs by even the smallest fraction each time you go out, you will certainly be keen to continue the trend during your next workouts. And when the day comes that your progress is negative, when you have slipped back a notch for any reason, your motivation for redoubling your efforts at the next chance will certainly ensure that you get back up to speed quickly.

Have I mentioned that having small, manageable goals within the context of your primary objective is a great method for keeping a positive intention and outlook on your fitness program? When you reach these smaller goals, fitness trackers allow you to visualize your victories and see your overall progress over smaller, connecting, time-frames. This is one marvelous technique that will keep you from being overwhelmed by always focusing on your main objective which may be realized only after another six months of regular workouts. Remember, your brain always guides you with positive intentions and thus secretly obliges you to stay on your program. I say "secretly" because you are not consistently aware of how your mind works to keep you on track. You will regularly be magically presented with benefits and rewards to staying focused, making it nearly impossible to skip a workout. If this sounds too hocus-pocus for you to accept as fact, ask yourself why so many athletes train so vigorously, often daily or even twice daily, for months at a time. Surely they must have other fun things to do, like going to the movies or dinners with friends, or just relaxing at home watching Netflix.

I can assure you, in their minds training hard every day is the most important and rewarding activity available. In fact, when they are not training, they are talking about training with their friends, planning the next challenging workout, and finally going to sleep early in order to be fully recharged for the next day's workout. An athlete's mind has been programmed to set goals and sub-goals, and his or her fitness gadget permits the athlete to receive the feedback necessary to feel great and progress. Can you consider that when you work out, that you *are* this athlete? You will feel wonderful about your progress, too.

Perhaps the most interesting advantage of wearing a fitness tracker, either in your smartphone or on your wrist, is the social experience. If you enjoy sharing achievements with your friends on Facebook or Instagram, then you will love your fitness tracker. You now have the opportunity of connecting with your friends and acquaintances through your tracker's website, or, directly on the app which you have downloaded to your smartphone.

As soon as your workout has ended, in the case of an app on your smartphone, or as soon as your wristband uploads the results to your computer, in the case of a physical device, the results are in turn uploaded into the Cloud. All your followers will instantly receive notifications of your results with various statistics pertaining to your activity. With running or cycling events, for instance, a map is normally generated showing the track that you covered, elevation gain, speeds, and so on. Conversely, when any of your connections completes a workout, you will receive a notification of their results. They can leave comments against each of your workouts as you can on theirs. You can imagine how the comments themselves can be quite entertaining.

Picture yourself after a grueling workout, refreshing yourself with your favourite beverage or an energy bar and suddenly your phone is buzzing with encouraging comments from your friends who have just read about your run, ride, swim or gym workout. It is fun and easy to stay in touch with your friends and acquaintances this way, even when they are training in different time zones or in different countries. The progress that your friends and other connections make is inspiring and will challenge you to keep up or surpass their accomplishments. The competition is friendly, the feedback is in real time, and as you will see for yourself, sharing your progress with others is a wonderful motivator. Our key is to maintain the motivation we need to stick to our training program and get into the best shape of our lives. These fun devices are indeed tremendous motivators.

Now let's have a quick look at the science: As I have written at the start of this book, being sufficiently motivated plays a pivotal role in whether you will be able to increase and maintain your physical activity levels. But not all forms of motivation are equally powerful. According to a prominent thesis in this area called *Self-Determination Theory*, a concept that grew out of researchers Edward Deci and Richard Ryan's work on motivation, three broad forms of motivation exist which vary in their quality. Let's understand them now.

When a person does something freely, willingly and with a positive attitude, it usually indicates higher motivational quality (autonomous motivation), whereas if a person does an activity mainly in response to demands or pressures of others, such as competition or comparison with them, this is indicative of lower motivational quality (controlled motivation). In contrast, a state of amotivation is when a person has no desire to take part in an activity at all.

Within this theory, greater motivation depends on three basic "needs": Autonomy, competence and relatedness. Autonomy is the need to feel a sense of ownership over your actions; competence is the need to feel adequately challenged and experience a sense of accomplishment; and relatedness is the need to feel connected to others and supported in your endeavors. Both autonomous (higher) and controlling (lower) forms of motivation can prompt changes in our behavior, but autonomous motivation is more enduring and beneficial in the longer term, particularly for physical activity, and unsurprisingly for weight loss, too. So, how can we enhance our autonomous motivation so that we look forward to and enjoy our workouts?

In a 2017 study carried out at the University of Glasgow, Craig Donnachie and Kate Hunt found how goal-setting and self-monitoring of progress by participants using fitness trackers supported the development of high-quality (autonomous) motivation for physical activity, during and after taking part in the study.

Some people who successfully made positive changes said they no longer used the tracker as their new, more active lifestyles had become second nature and being active in their day-to-day lives had become part of their identity. Others still used their self-monitoring devices because they enjoyed keeping track of how active they were and it helped them sustain their increased activity levels.

Now, our question is answered: Clearly, in the case of many people, wearing a fitness tracker allows them to review and measure their progress and boosts their feelings of self-confidence. Fitness trackers are a fantastic boon for many people. Downloading an app that your friends are already using is fast, easy and free. It may be all you need to help you jumpstart your training program and achieve your goals while enjoying the journey along the way.

# Strategy Seven: Listen to music

A number of people believe that they get a better workout when they listen to music while training. Your favorite workout tunes may act as natural pain relievers and help you to move faster, or lift heavier weights, without you even realizing it. Listening to music while exercising can release feel-good chemicals in the brain – such as dopamine and serotonin – that may boost your mood, make you less tired, and even dull pain, scientists say.

Neuroscientist and author of *This Is Your Brain on Music,* Dr. Daniel Levitin, explains that there are two possible mechanisms, both of which contribute to a better workout. Either music acts as a distractor or as a mood enhancer. Distractors are known to modulate pain levels. I have read that combat soldiers, policemen and firemen don't always realize that they have been seriously wounded or even shot until after the excitement of the moment is over. If you plan on having a brutal workout one day, then also plan on using some kind of distractor to help you successfully complete your effort.

In their book, *The Social and Applied Psychology of Music*, Adrian North and David Hargreaves suggested that music distracts from fatigue endured during exercise through competing stimuli. It is easier to forget about fatigue when a song you enjoy is distracting you. Music that you enjoy will cause the release of mood-enhancing chemicals in the brain which, in turn, raises the pain threshold. You may have heard about the feel-good hormone serotonin which is produced by the brain when you listen to music that you enjoy. Everyone has at least once seen a teenager with headphones playing the air guitar, completely unaware of all those around watching him, as he imagines himself making or playing the music he is listening to on his imaginary guitar.

As serotonin and other hormones do increase in our brains while listening to music when we exercise, then we will be put in a better mood naturally and feel great. Just as you may get excited about watching the next episode of your favourite Netflix series, you will be eager to get to your next workout or spinning class thanks to your mood-enhancing music. Now you can understand why cardio classes are often overflowing with participants, standing room only, if you'll pardon the pun. The instructors with the best music always have the most crowded classes and notably the fittest members. These fit members are not more attracted than other people to good music. Rather, it is the great music that stimulates them to unwittingly push themselves to their limits and often beyond. You may inadvertently have felt this intense energy yourself as you walk by a spinning class in progress, hearing the music turned up, feeling the bass vibrations in your body, and witnessing the vigorous efforts made by those inside. The result is the same whether you bring your own tunes and headphones to your workout, or you participate in a group class with music supplied. I should note that cycling outdoors with headphones or earbuds is risky business and outlawed in some jurisdictions.

The research is still better for you who prefer an endurance-oriented fitness program. Studies show that listening to music while working out can help you regulate and maintain an exercise pace that you may have trouble with, without music. Apparently there is a link between music tempo and exercise performance. In one study, cyclists tended to work harder while listening to faster-paced music. Another found identical results for runners. In both cases, the tempo of the music made it feel easier to synchronize strides or pedaling at a faster pace, seemingly with less effort.

According to the majority of studies, and there are many linking music to motivation and performance, the beat of the music surreptitiously urges your body to work harder to match the music's rhythm. If you want to maximize your improvement, always choose a selection of tunes whose beat is slightly faster than your usual pace. The process takes effect in the background. You will be unaware that you are running or cycling faster unless you specifically concentrate on your speed. Few of us focus exclusively on our pace as we tend to fall into some kind of trance while running, cycling or during other similar aerobic exercises. The rhythmic nature of the activity naturally permits our minds to wander, daydream and otherwise lose track of time.

Listening to music while exercising doesn't just relieve boredom – it can help improve the quality of your workout by increasing your stamina and putting you in a better mood. The effects of music lead to higher than expected levels of endurance, power or strength. This will result in approaching and ultimately achieving your fitness goal sooner. Your accelerated progress becomes a powerful motivator to stick with your program and continue improving.

There is yet one more benefit to creating your own exercise playlist. Researchers Leon Szmedra and David Bacharach found that "some of the by-product molecules of high level exercise, such as acidosis and elevated hormones (which contribute to fatigue), may be dampened by music, thus enhancing performance." Finally, once your workout is over, listening to music that is normally reserved for a yoga class will help you to relax and perhaps avoid post-workout muscle soreness. Just as an upbeat tempo can stimulate you to exercise with more intensity, so does relaxing music help you to slow down and recover contentedly from your challenging workout.

It is no wonder that more and more people can be seen wearing stylish headphones or wireless earbuds in the gym or while running in the streets. As with the other strategies, any tactic used for enjoying your workouts is an excellent stimulus to train hard and get into the best shape of your life.

# Bonus strategy: Keep a training log or journal

Studies consistently show us that when we write things down we are more likely to achieve our objective. Getting into the best shape of your life is hard work. It is important to train frequently to your limit, so that both your cardiovascular system and your muscles will respond naturally by increasing their capacity and strength. A reliable motivator is to see your progress on a continual basis, not only in the mirror, but also in your training log.

Let's use a very simple example: You have decided to challenge yourself, get into shape and run a 10-km race in one hour or faster in a specific race which takes place in six months. Today, you cannot jog 15 minutes without stopping to catch your breath; running (and walking) 10 km will take you almost 85 minutes. You join a running group at the local athletic shoes store for motivation, camaraderie, support and training tips. You learn about interval training, long runs, hill work and technique. Remarkably, it's a lot of fun and you are making new friends as a bonus.

The group meets two evenings a week plus weekends. They break into packs of faster runners, intermediate runners and slower runners. You find your group and start running three times a week. Now, after every run, locate your training log and write down the date, then your distance, your time, the weather and any other details that matter to you. After only a few weeks, you'll have a lot of entries and you can easily begin to see your improvement.

It's very satisfying to see for yourself how your speeds have been increasing, not necessarily every day, but over time. You note that you are walking less and running more. You read in your comments that you are less often out of breath, that you are keeping up with the rest of the pack, no longer trailing behind. Your motivation to continue toward your objective, to run that 10-km race, is very strong. Nothing will get in your way of crossing the finish line in under one hour.

Writing down our goals, whether running faster on the track or lifting heavier weights in the gym, focuses our minds on success. Reading about our progress motivates us to push ourselves and excel. Now that you have read about these successful strategies, your work has just begun. Anybody can choose today to get into the best shape of his or her life. Make that choice now and start today. You deserve to feel marvelous and look awesome, don't you?.